HAPPY, HEALTHY TEETH!

A Guide to Children's Dental Health

Anubha Sacheti, DMD

Deidre Callanan, RDH, DC, MPH

Nancy Topping-Tailby, LICSW

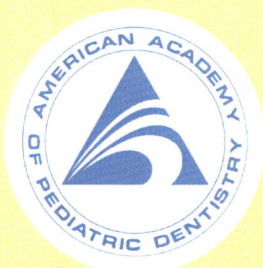

The information presented in this book has been reviewed by AAPD and found to be consistent with the current science related to oral care for children.

Pictures by Glenn Weinreb, Billie Wong and Portrait Simple in Chestnut Hill, MA

Thank you to Callum Douglass and Hiran Kuru.

Design by Melissa Greenberg

Printed by the HF Group in the USA

HAPPY, HEALTHY TEETH!

Copyright 2011 © by Massachusetts Head Start Association, Inc.

All rights reserved. Except as permitted under the U.S. Copyright Act of 1976, no part of this publication may be reproduced, distributed, or transmitted in any form or by any means, or stored in a database or retrieval system, without the prior written permission of Massachusetts Head Start Association, Inc.

ISBN: 978-1-60414-455-0 (hardcover)

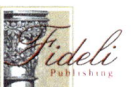

Published by Fideli Publishing, Inc.

www.FideliPublishing.com

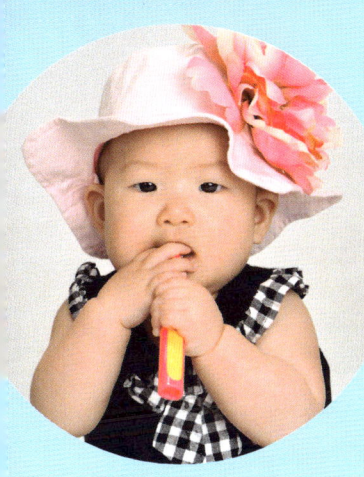 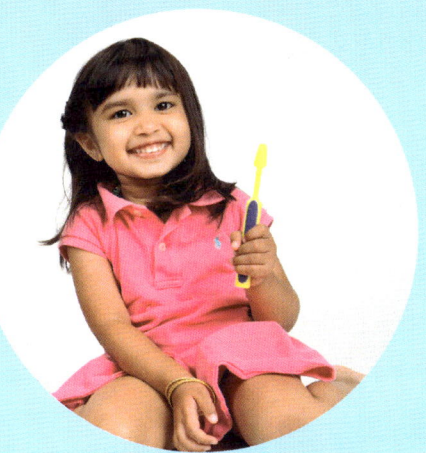 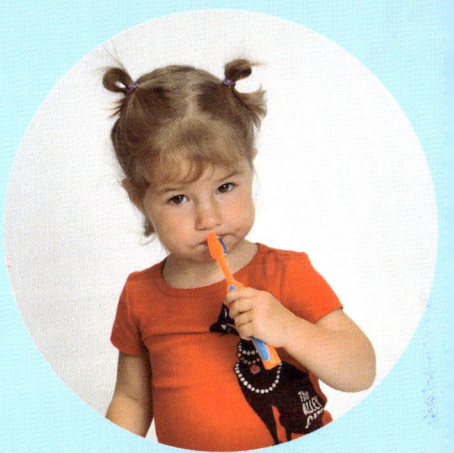

This book is dedicated to Head Start children, families and program staff. School readiness depends on children's healthy development, and healthy development includes oral health!

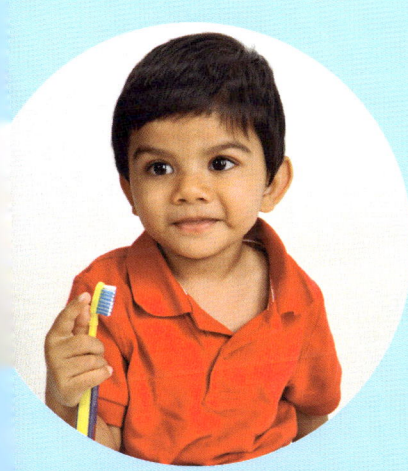 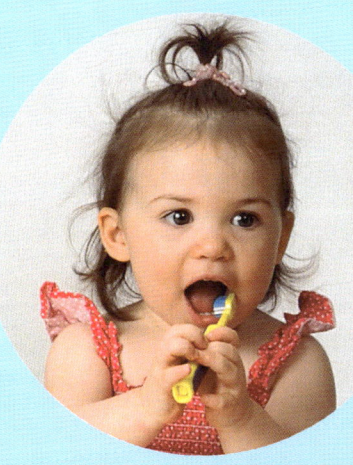 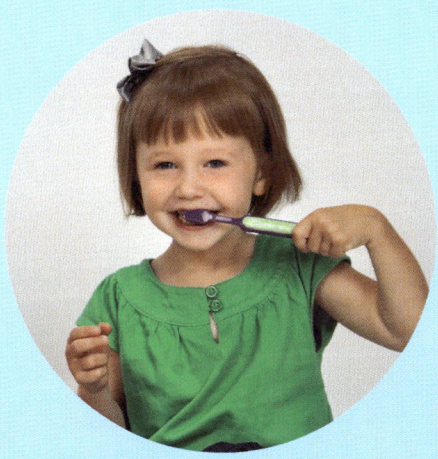

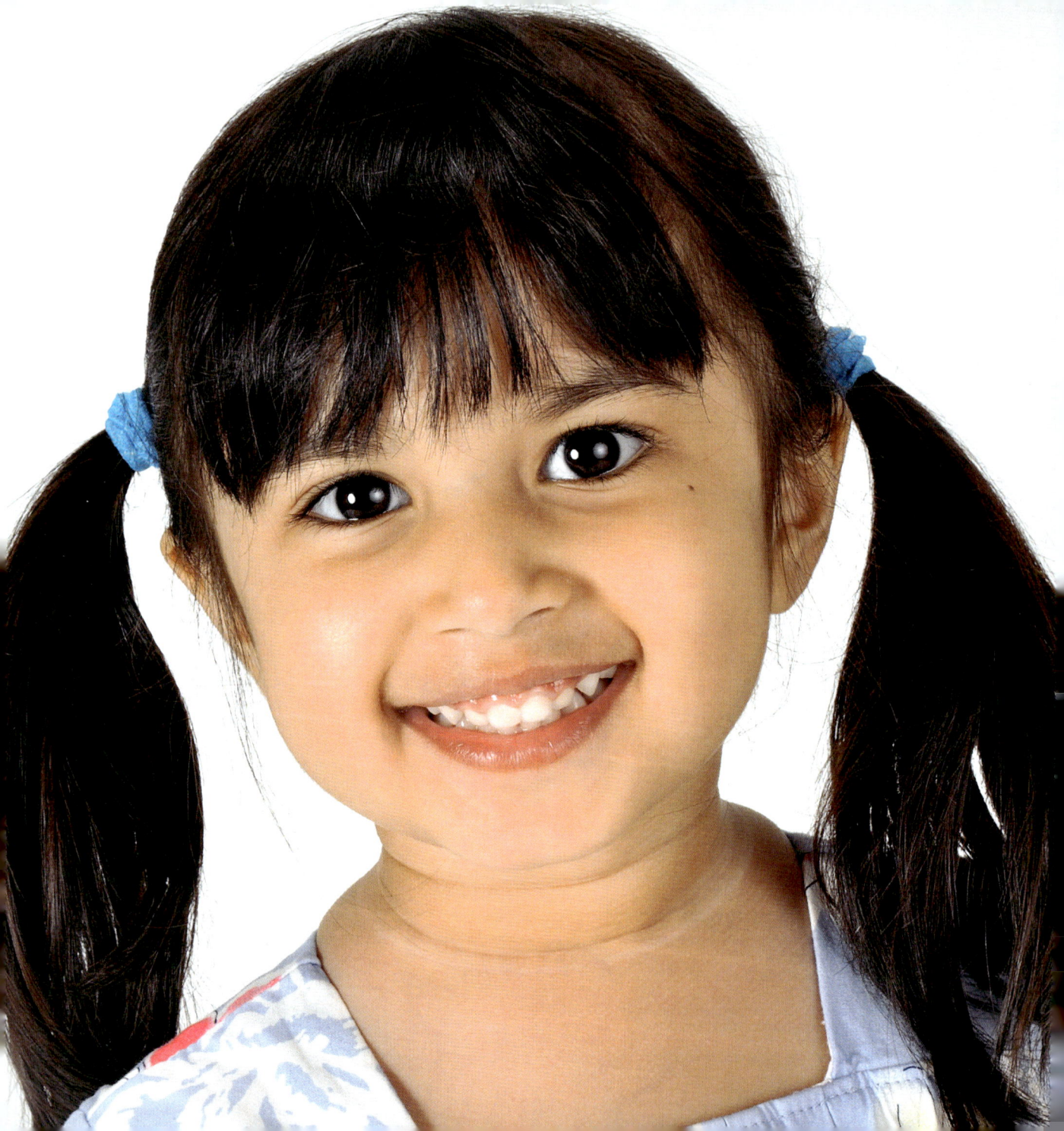

Meet 2 year old Aleena.
Her teeth are shiny and bright.

Her Momma brushes her teeth both morning and night.

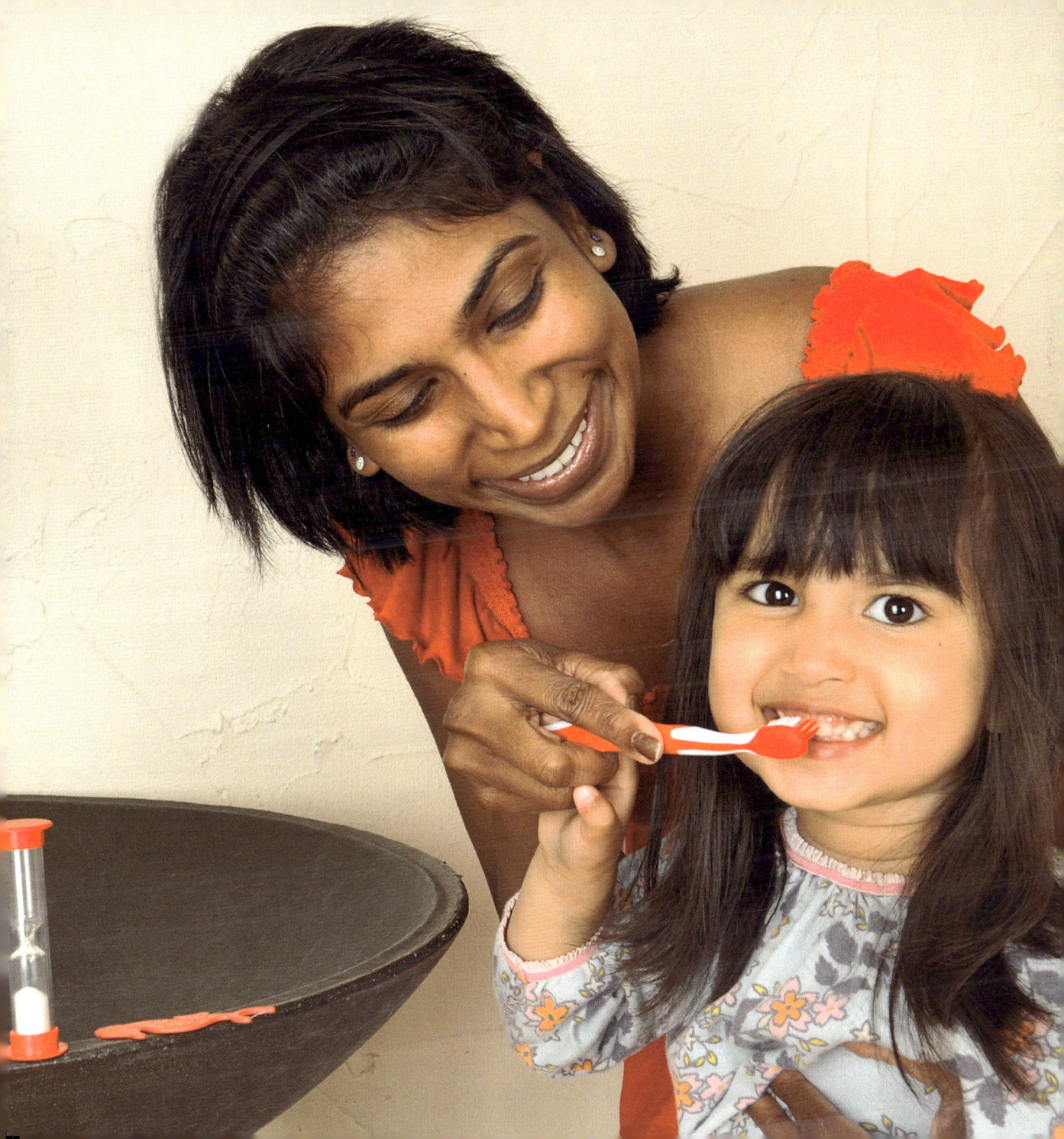

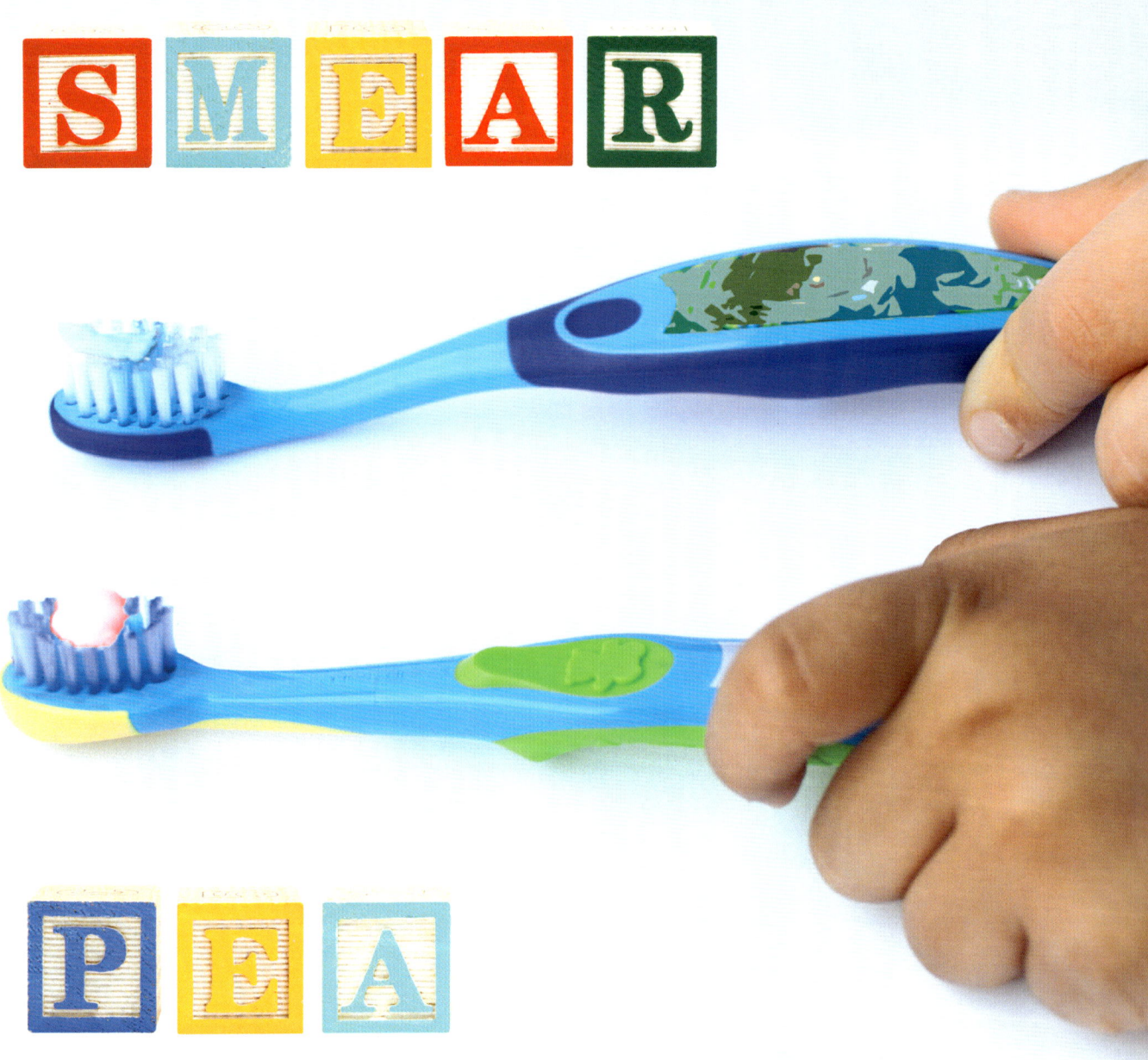

Toothpaste with fluoride keeps teeth healthy and white. For babies, a tiny smear is just right.*

When kids are two, a pea-sized amount will do.

*Consult your dentist for more information regarding the use of fluoride toothpaste for children younger than 2.

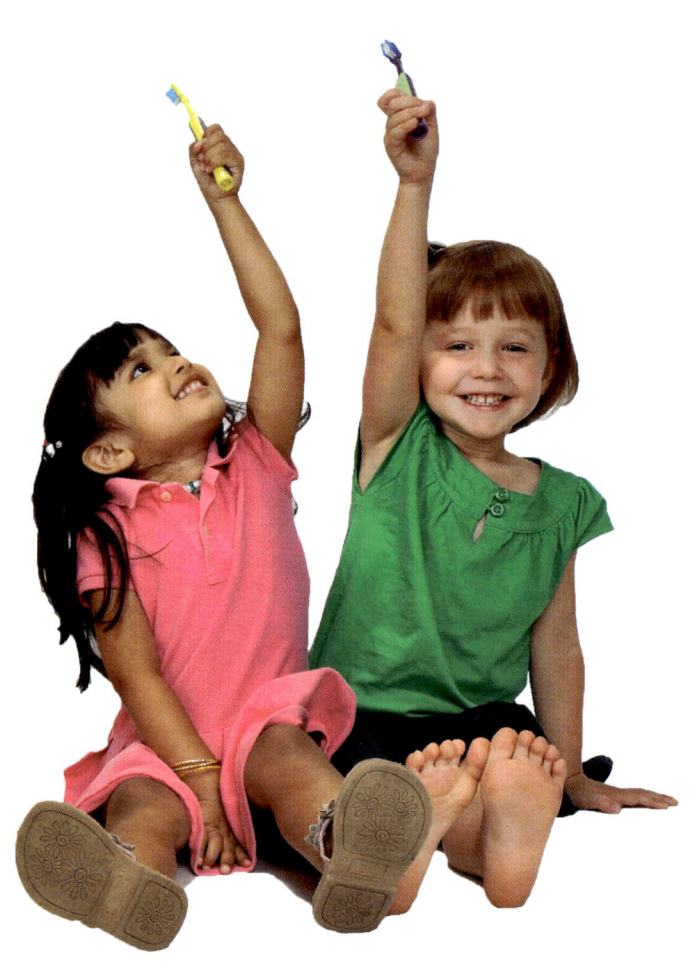
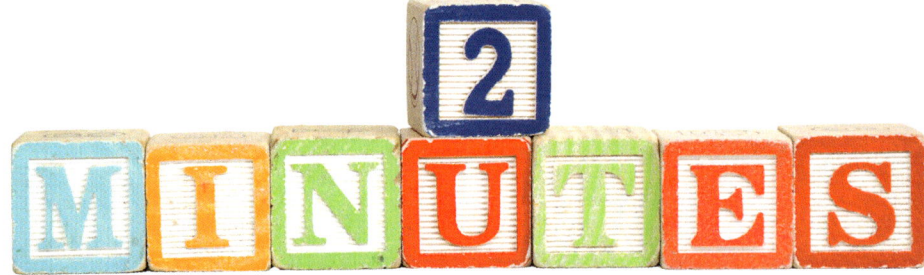

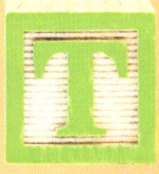wo minutes of brushing helps teeth stay strong.

Set a timer or sing a song, and it won't seem too long.

Whether you're a grown-up or still very young, finish by brushing all over your tongue.

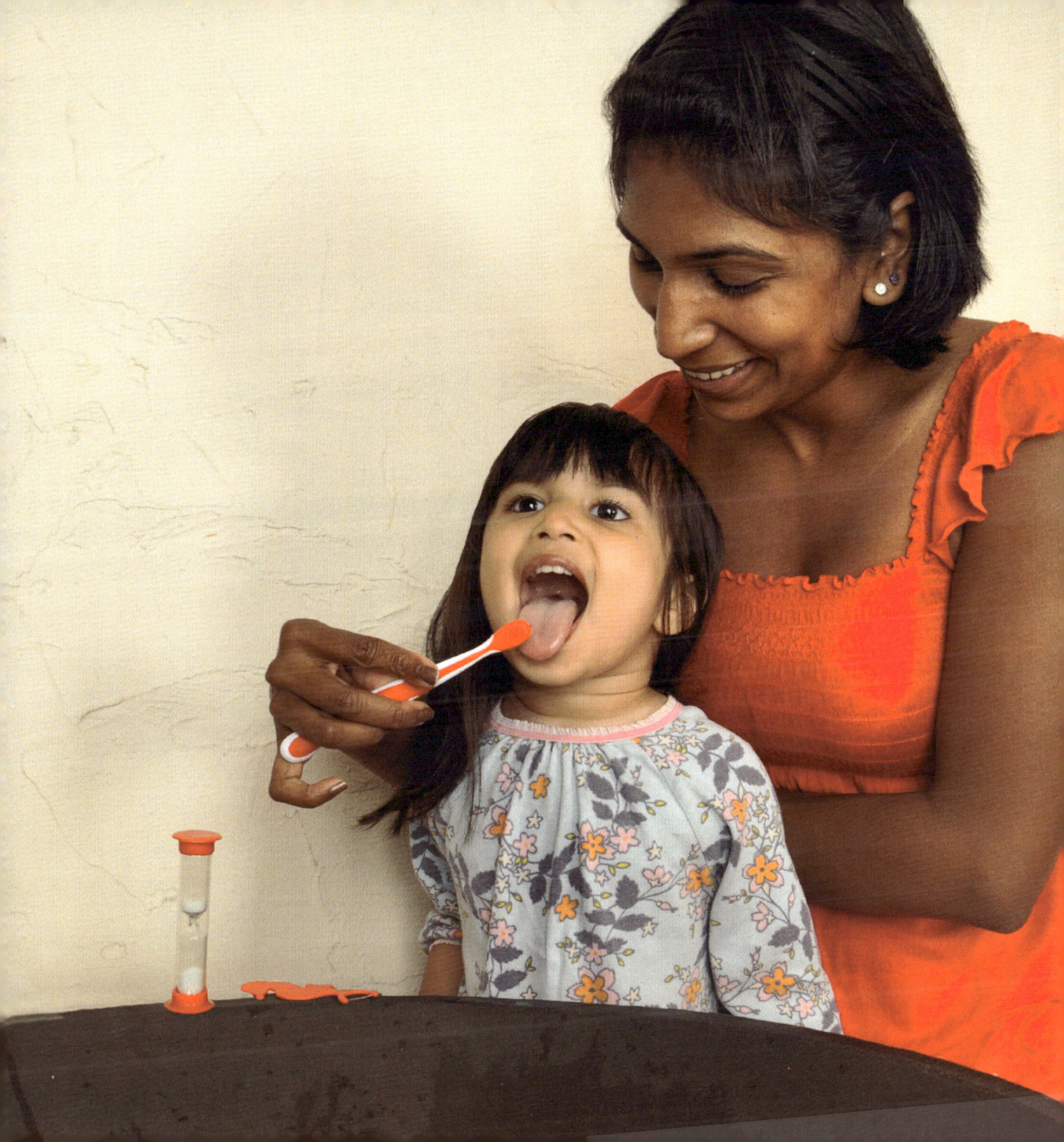

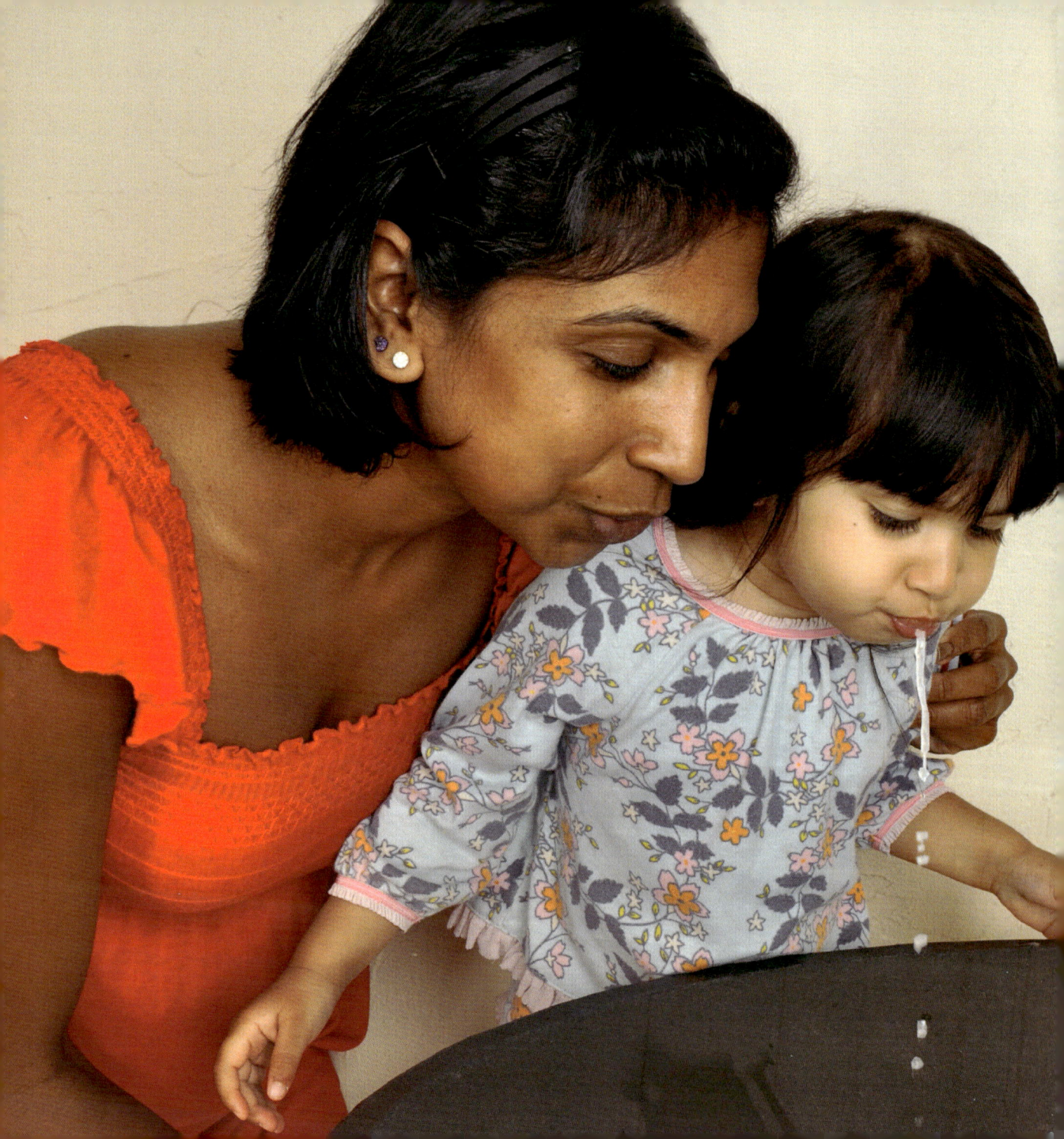

Spit out when you're done, but don't rinse the toothpaste away. It's good for your teeth while you sleep and play.

Don't share your toothbrush.
It's not a toy! It's just for you -
not another girl or boy.

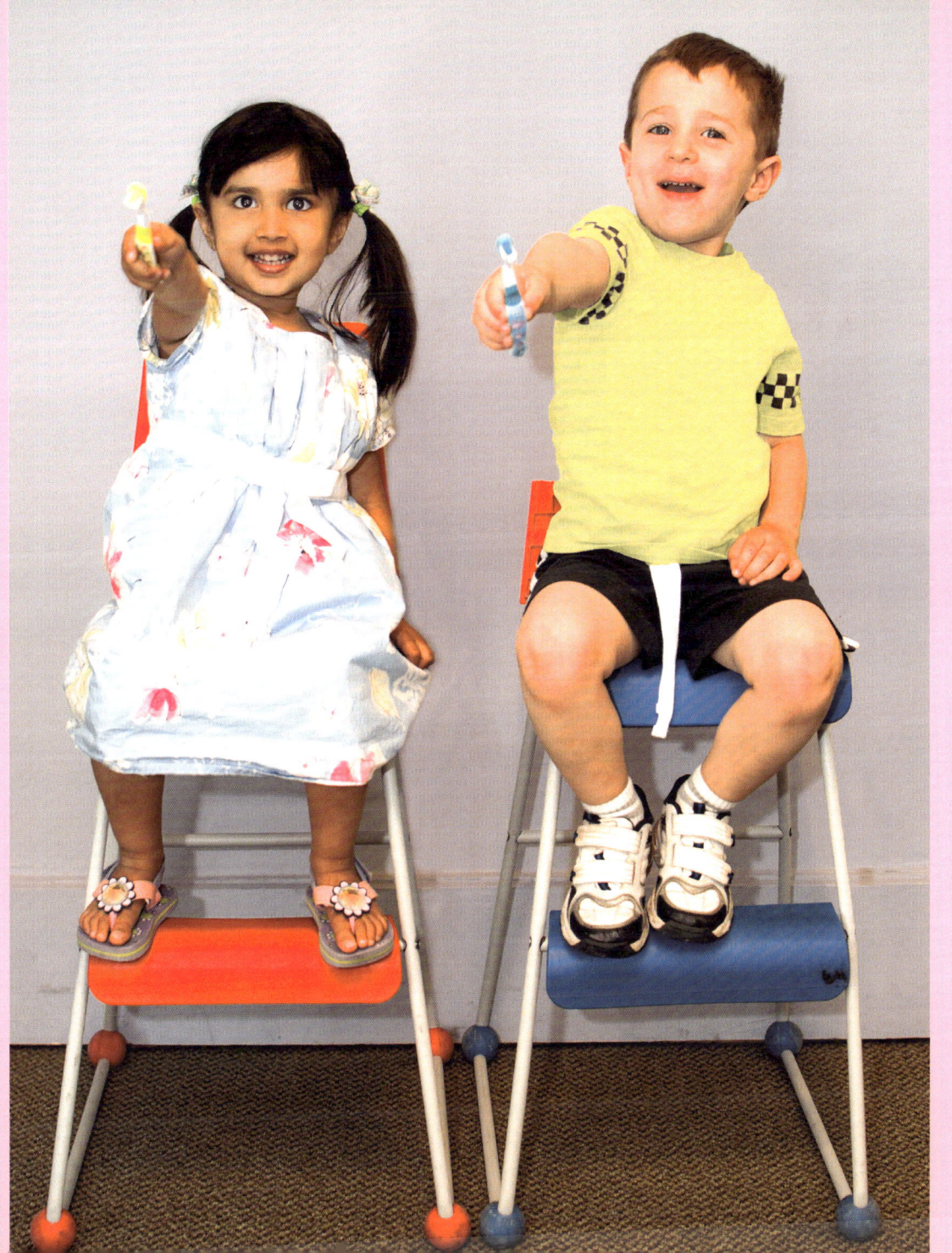

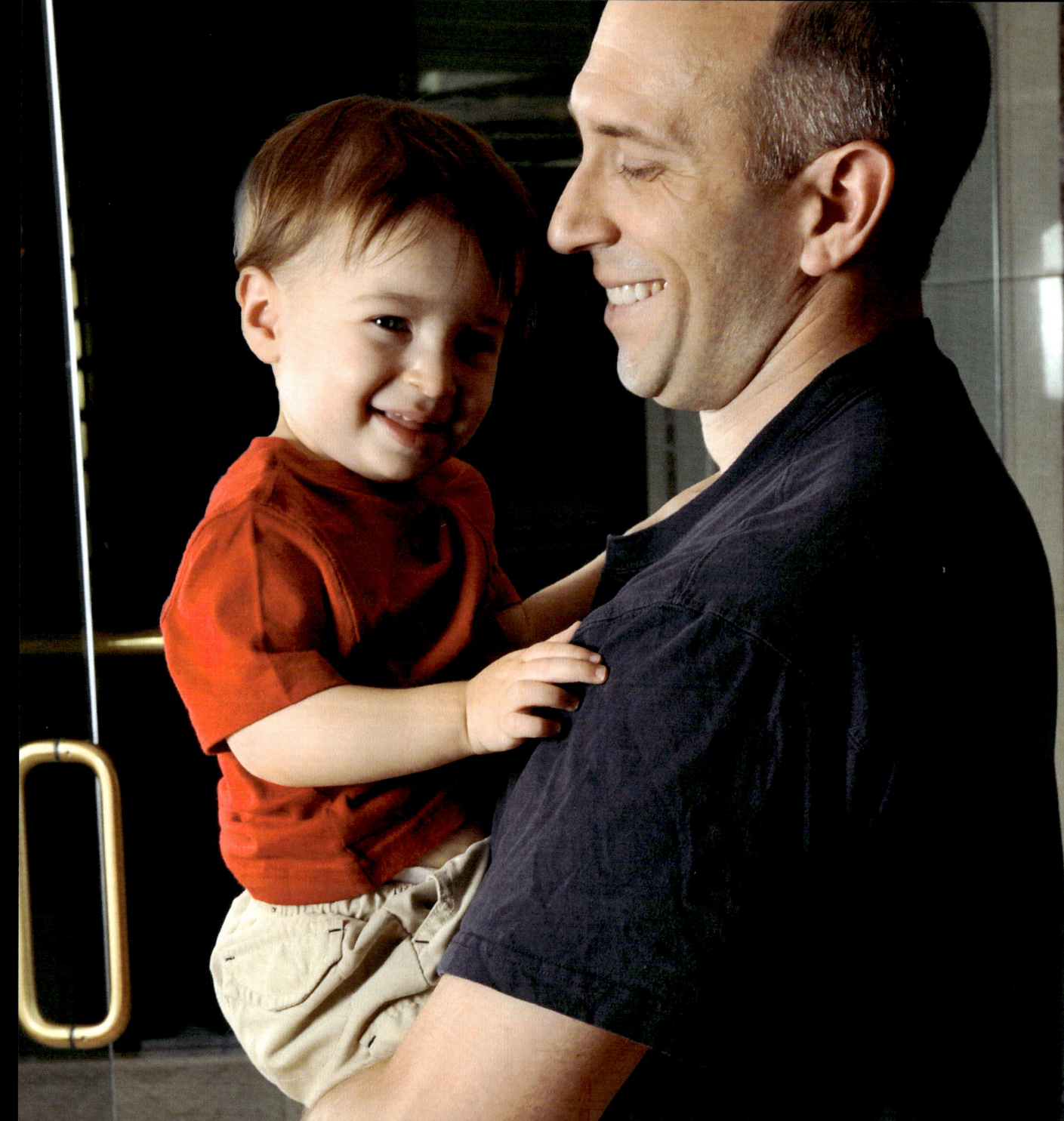

Going to the dentist is so much fun. All kids should visit by the time they're one.

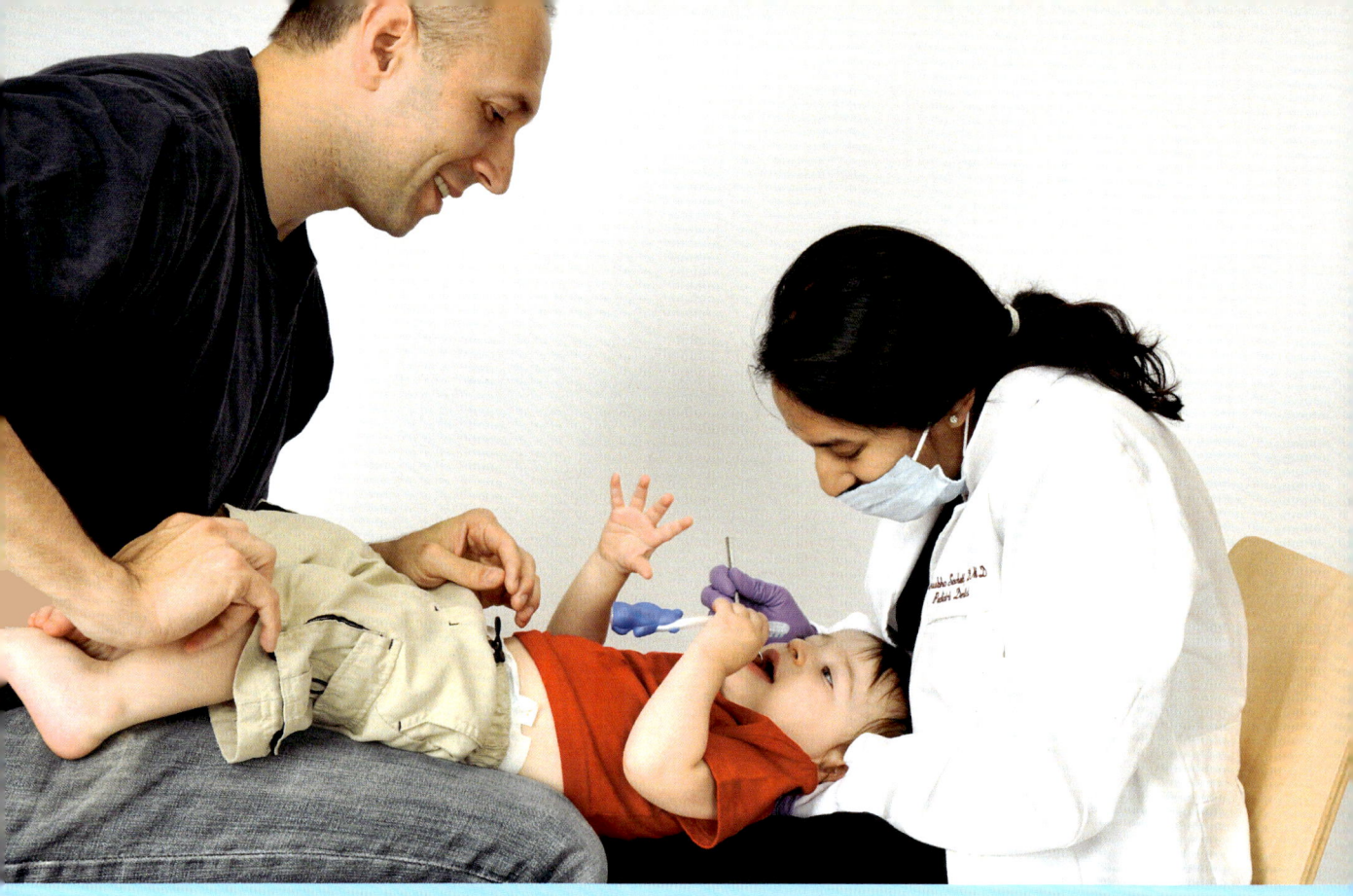

Babies lay back with their mouths open wide. The dentist has a mirror to see inside.

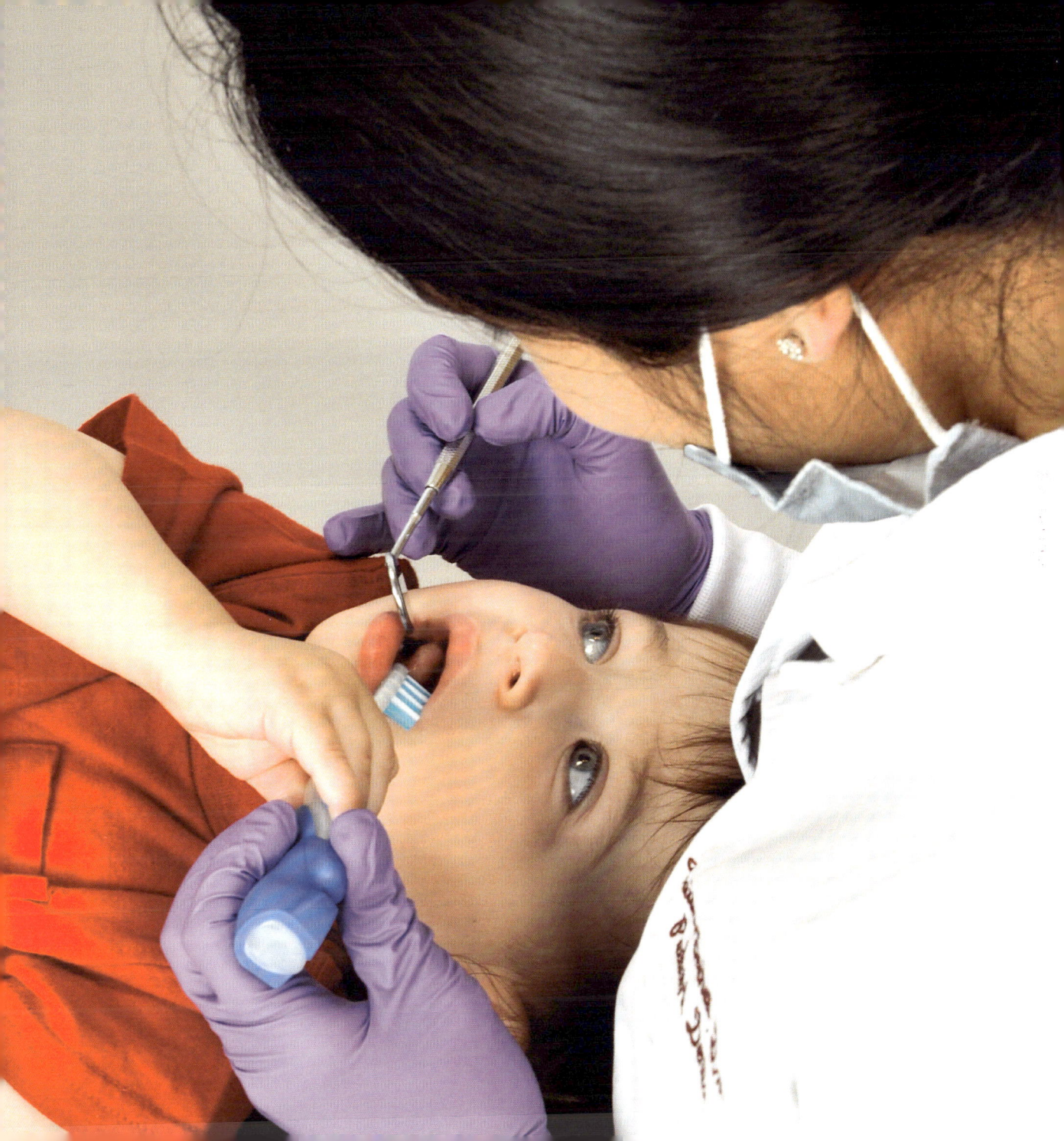

There's a big chair for Aleena to sit. The dentist counts her teeth to see how they fit.

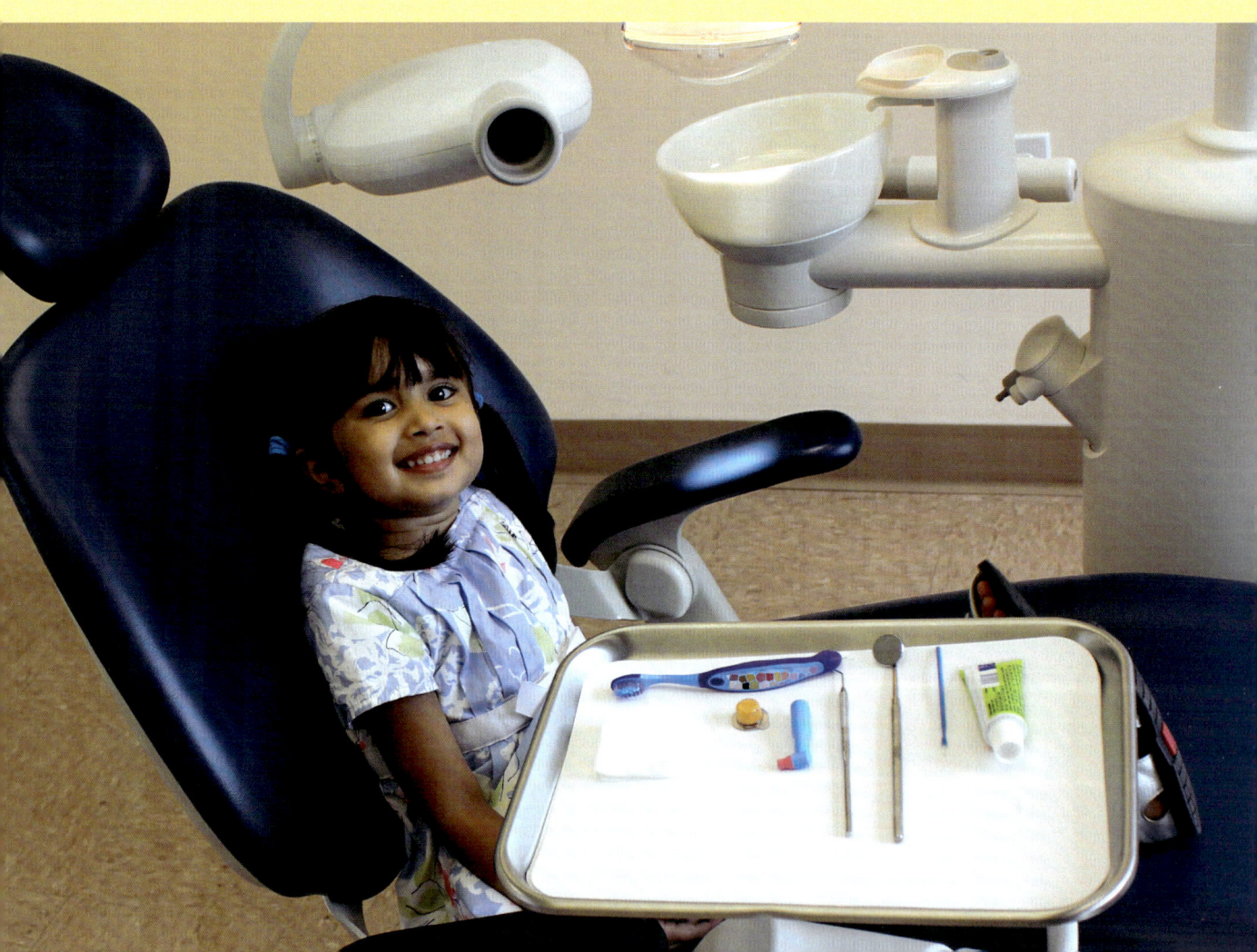

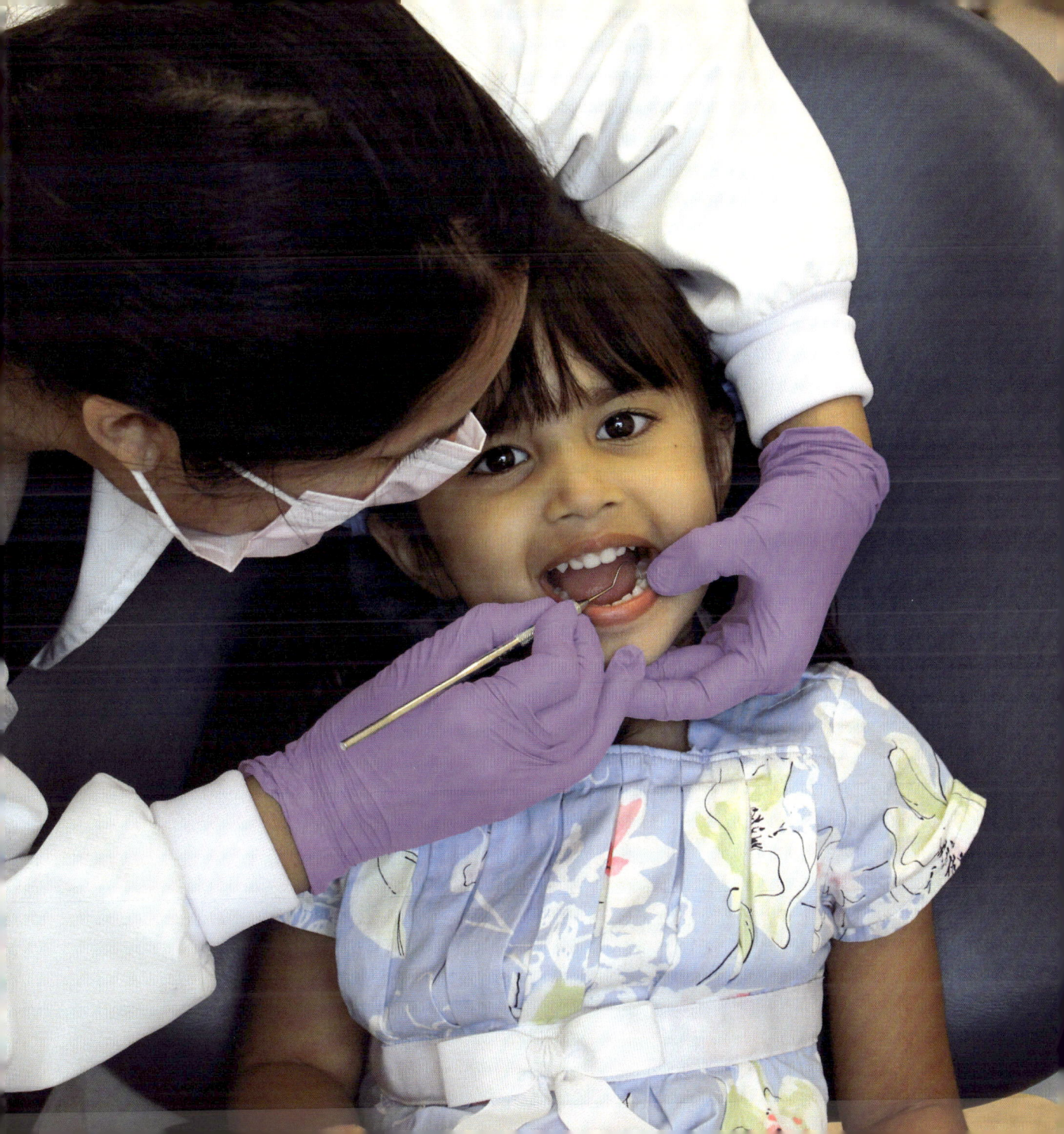

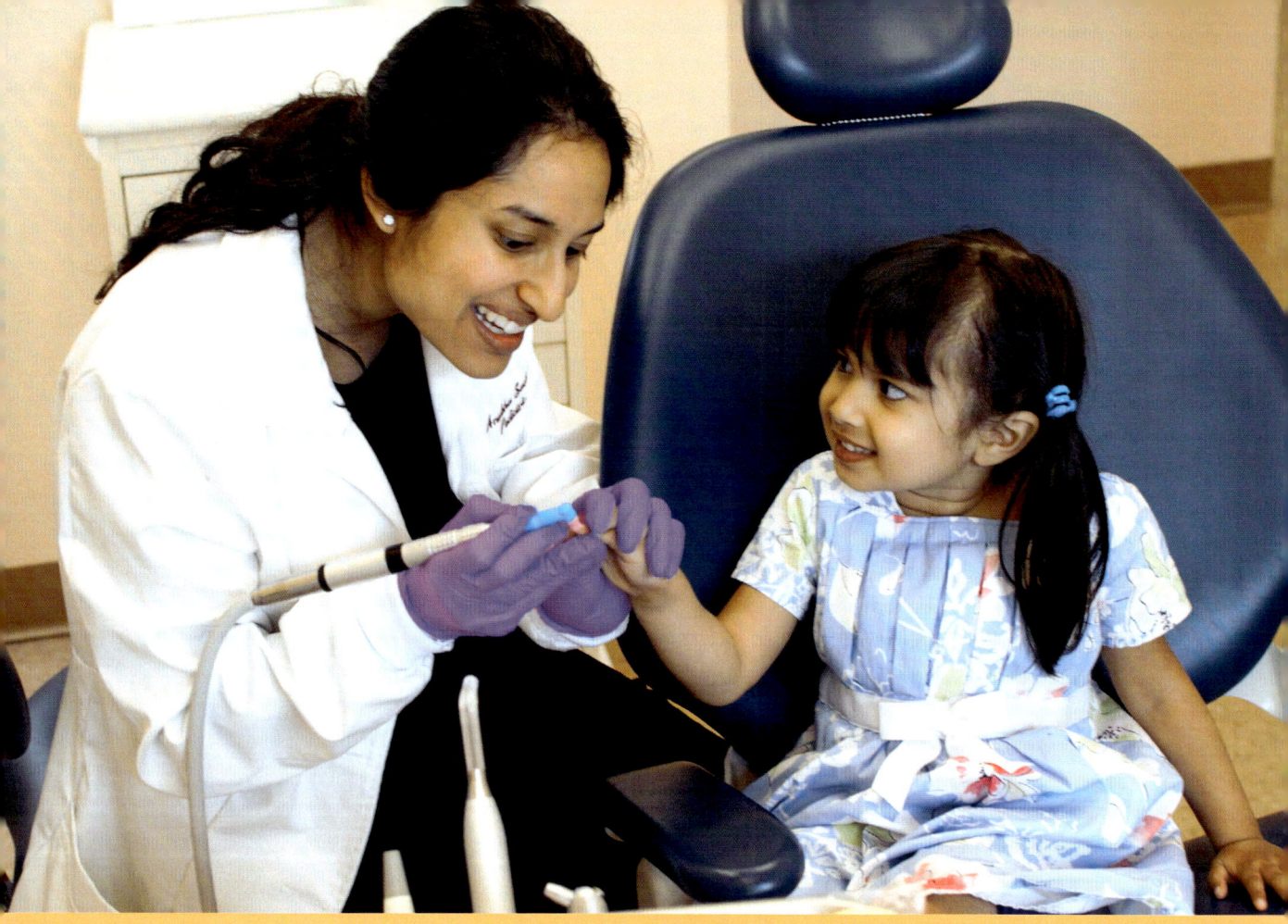

A special toothbrush tickles her teeth and cleans them just right.

Then on goes the fluoride to keep them sparkly and bright.

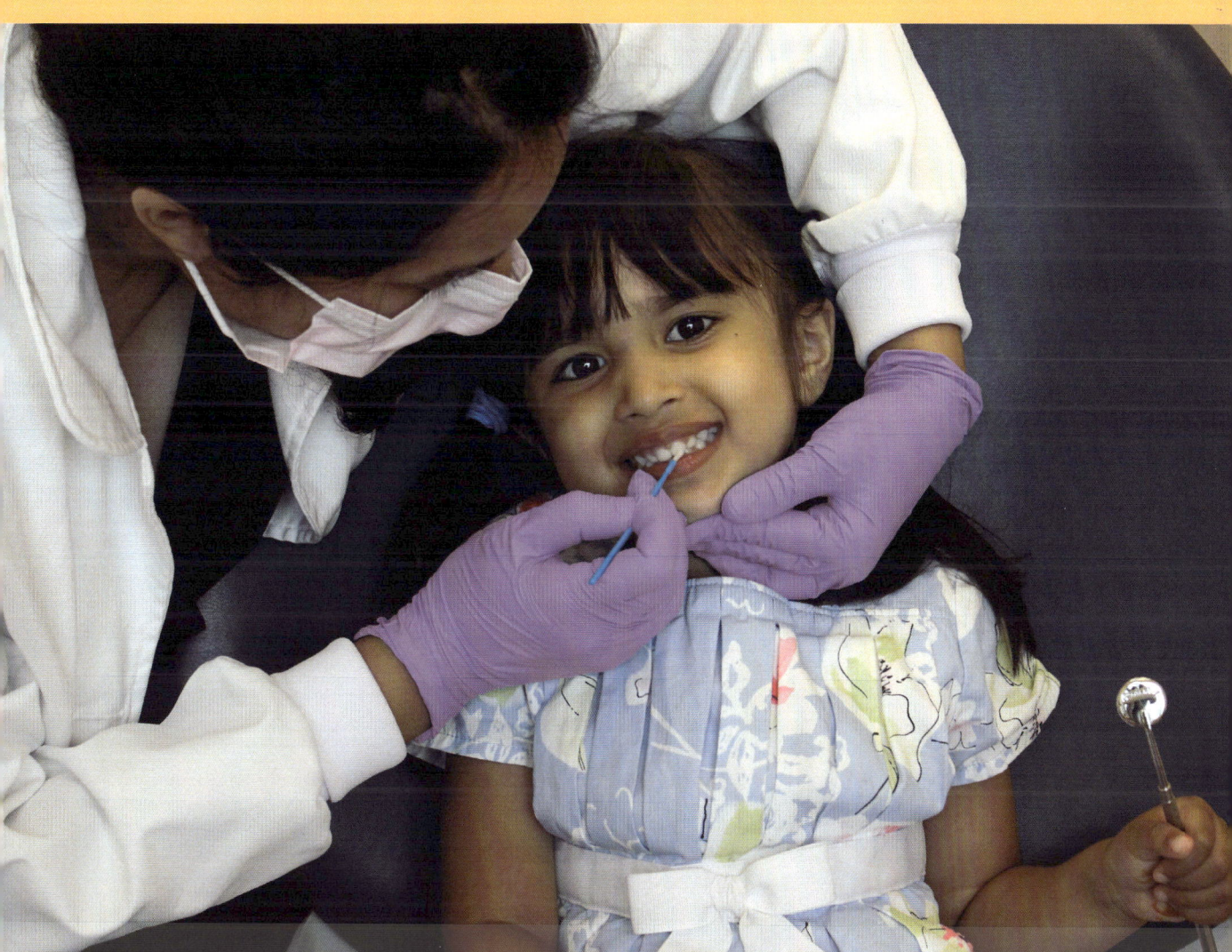

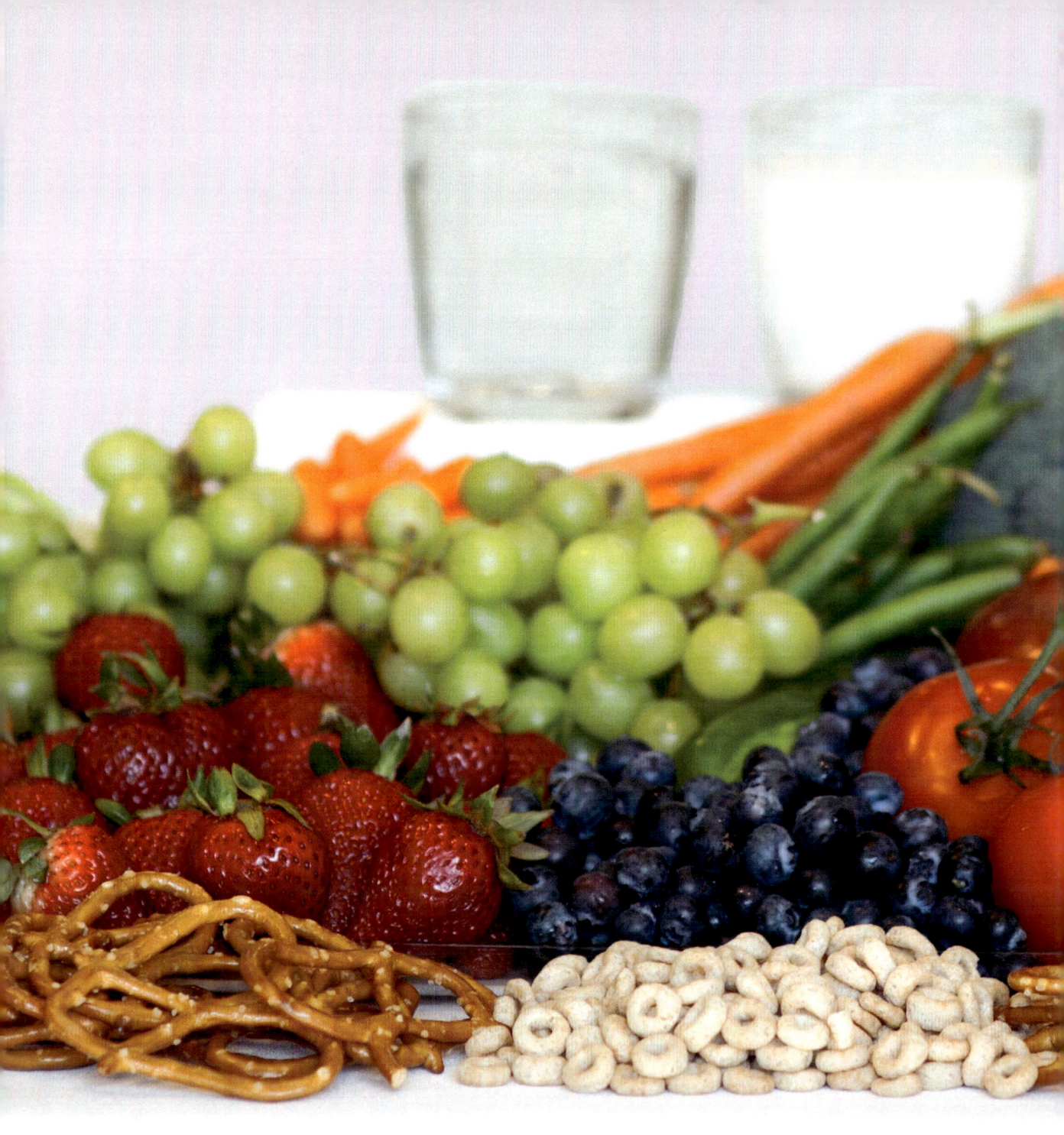

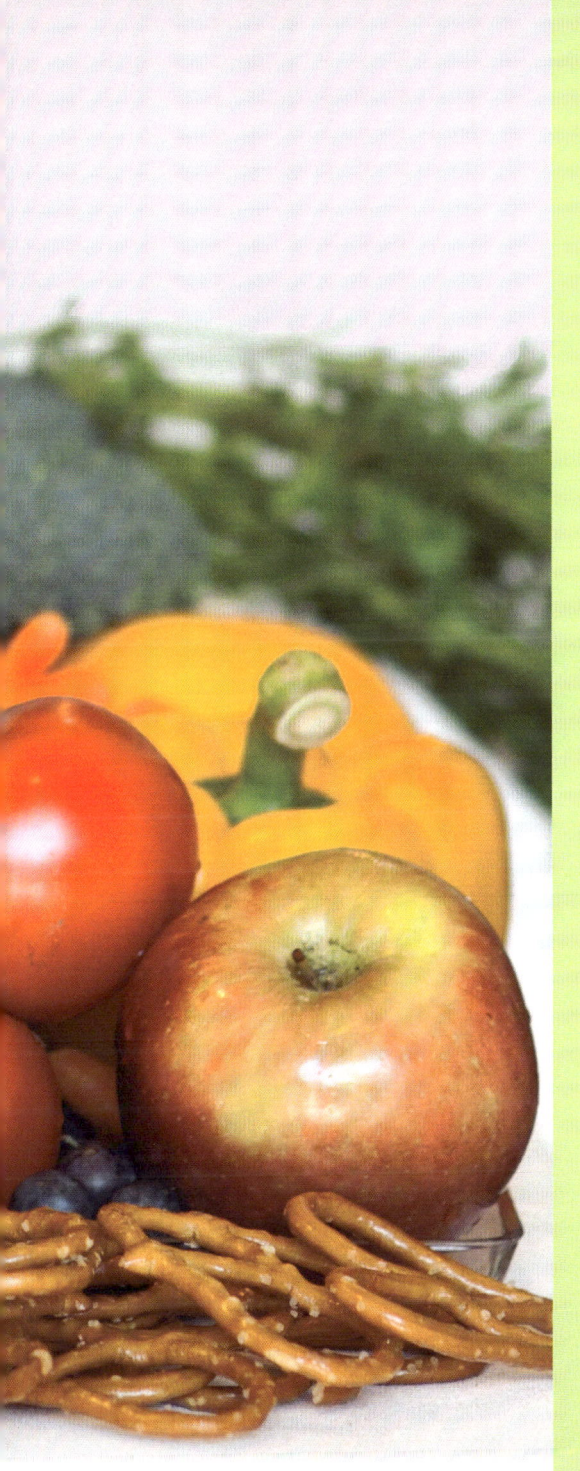

Drink milk or water. Healthy food with no added sugar is best.

At bedtime, no food or drinks after brushing - it's time to rest!

Great job, Aleena! Let's choose a prize today.

Here's a new toothbrush. Momma will help you use it twice a day!

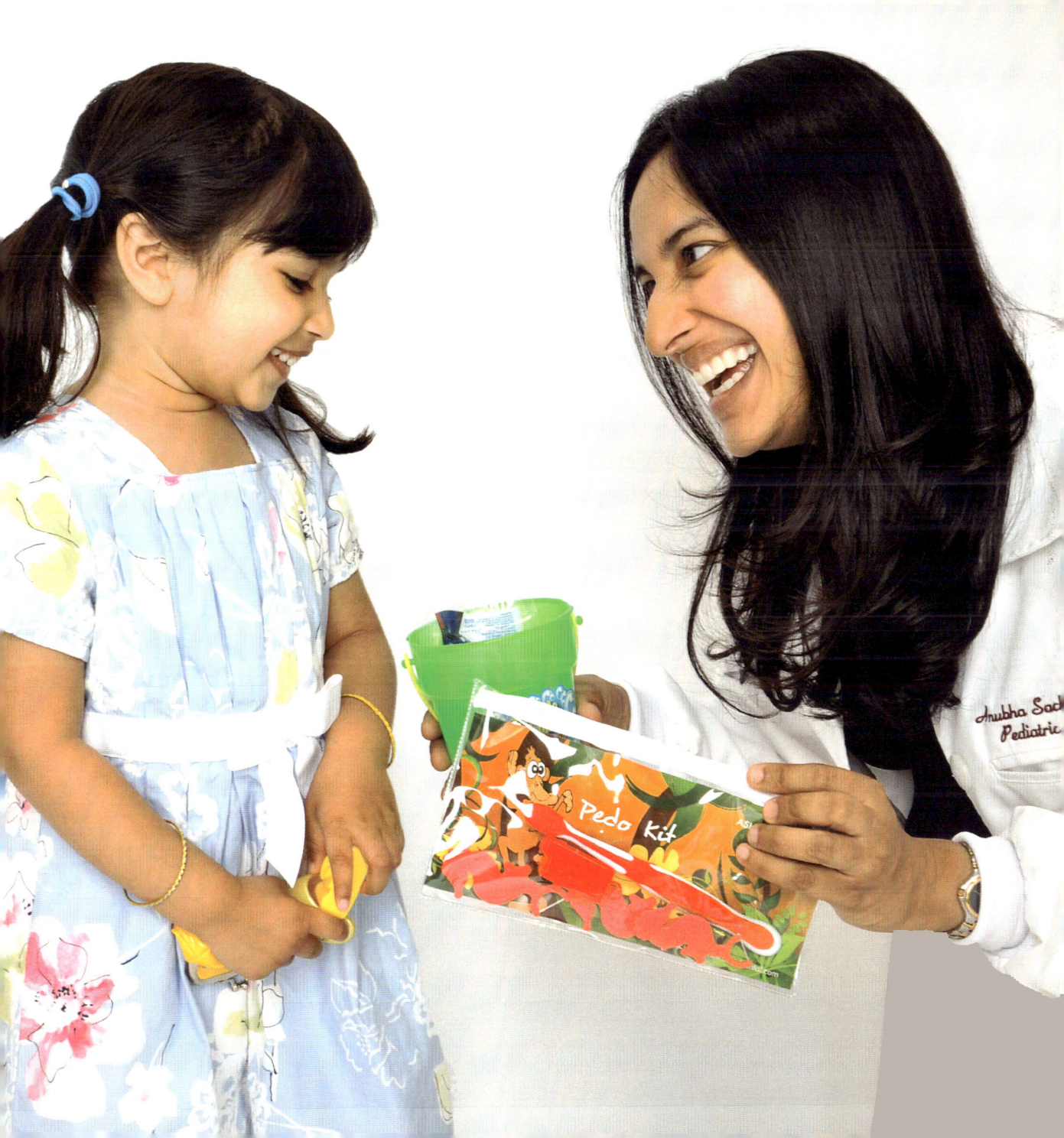

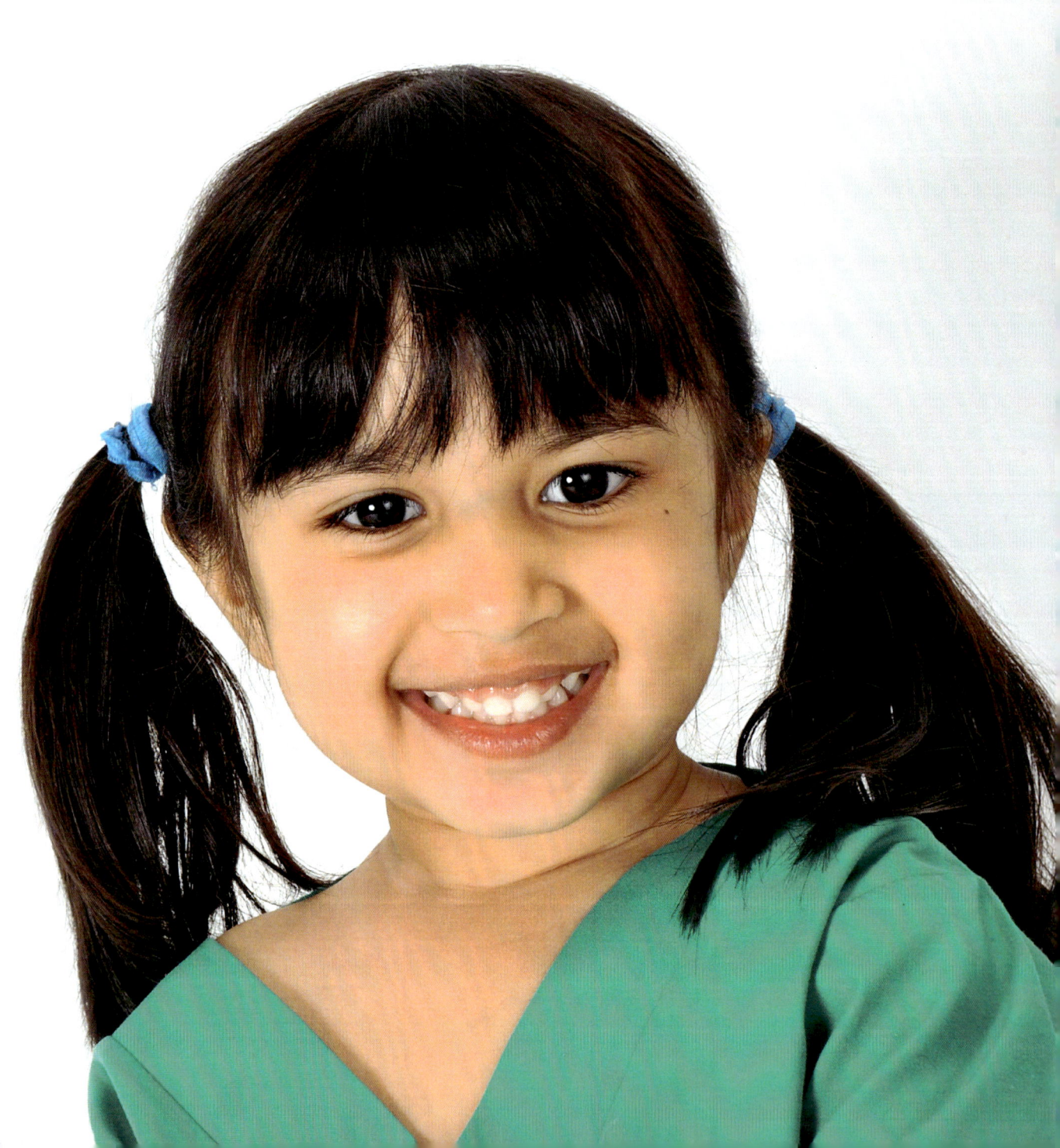

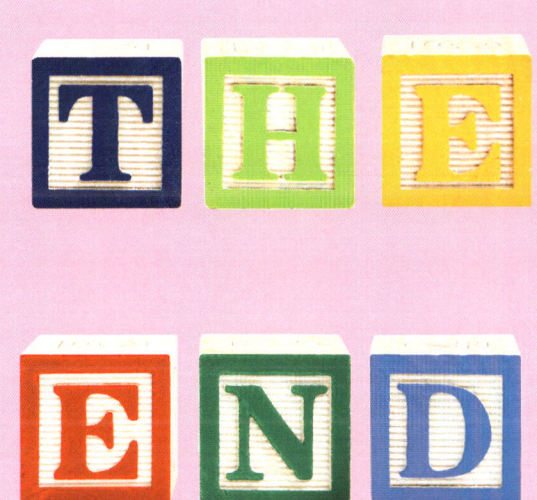

Family Guide / Note from Authors

Our goal is to help children care for their teeth with your help and to prepare them for the 1st dental visit.

We know that families are very diverse. Please change "Momma" to Dada, Grandma or your name when reading this book to your child.

Tooth Brushing Recommendations:

[1] Parents should brush their children's teeth until age 7 or 8.

[2] All children should use toothpaste with fluoride (it makes teeth strong & prevents cavities).

[3] Brush teeth for 2 minutes with a soft bristled toothbrush using only a smear of toothpaste for children under two and a pea-sized amount for children over the age of two.

[4] Remember to use a new brush when bristles are bent or broken.

[5] Don't let your children rinse after brushing. Water washes away the fluoride.

[6] Don't eat or drink after children's nighttime brushing. It's time for bed!!

Additional Brushing Tips for Toddlers:

- Give your child a tooth brush to hold while you use a 2nd brush to clean the teeth.
- Brush in front of a mirror so your child can watch.
- Brush after bathing, while your child is wrapped in a towel.

Food & Drink recommendations:

[1] Good foods & drinks lead to good teeth.

[2] During the day the best drinks are plain milk & water. Avoid juice & soda which contain sugar. Sugar causes cavities.

[3] Eat snacks during snack time - not all day long.

[4] Some medicines have a lot of sugar so brush or rinse afterwards.

Recommendations for Going to the Dentist:

Cavities are a disease and need to be treated. If cavities aren't treated, they can cause pain and serious infections. Tooth decay affects more children than any other childhood disease. It is five times more common than asthma!

Starting with pregnancy, moms need to take care of their teeth too because bacteria on the teeth can be passed from caregiver to child. One way to make sure that your child has healthy teeth is for everyone in the family to make good oral health care part of the daily routine.

The American Academy of Pediatric Dentistry recommends that children see the dentist as soon as they get their first tooth and no later than 12 months of age. Look for a dentist who can provide a comprehensive "dental home" and will see your child for both routine and emergency care if needed.

Children may cry a little bit when the dentist looks in their mouth. Crying actually makes it easier for the dentist to take a quick look inside the child's mouth! The dentist can see if your child has early signs of cavities. There are many things your dentist can do, with your help, to help stop cavities from happening.

To keep your child healthy, children need regular visits to the dentist at least every 6 months, just like they need regular visits to the doctor. If you don't have a dentist:

- Ask your child's pediatrician for help;

- Contact your state dental association;

- Check the website of the American Academy of Pediatric Dentistry http://www.aapd.org to find a pediatric dentist in your area; or

- Check the website of the American Dental Association http://www.ada.org to locate a general dentist.

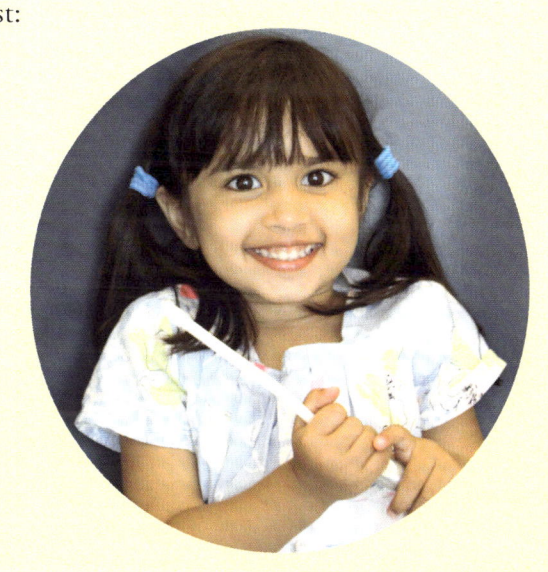

Acknowledgements

We received invaluable encouragement, support, and guidance over the many months it took to create this book.

We would like to thank the DentaQuest Foundation for generously funding this project.

The DentaQuest Foundation (dentaquestfoundation.org) is committed to optimal oral health for all Americans through its support of prevention and access to affordable care, and through its partnerships with funders, policymakers and community leaders.

We would also like to thank Dr. Joanna Douglass, BDS, DDS, our technical consultant.

We received valuable input from the members of the MA Early Childhood Oral Health Consortium and especially want to acknowledge Dr. Corinna Culler, Dr. Michelle Dalal, Kathy Dolan, Ellen Factor, Nancy Johnson, Dr. Man Wai Ng, and Maureen Vosburg for their comments. Thank you as well to the Massachusetts Dental Society and Jan Silverman from the American Academy of Pediatric Dentistry.

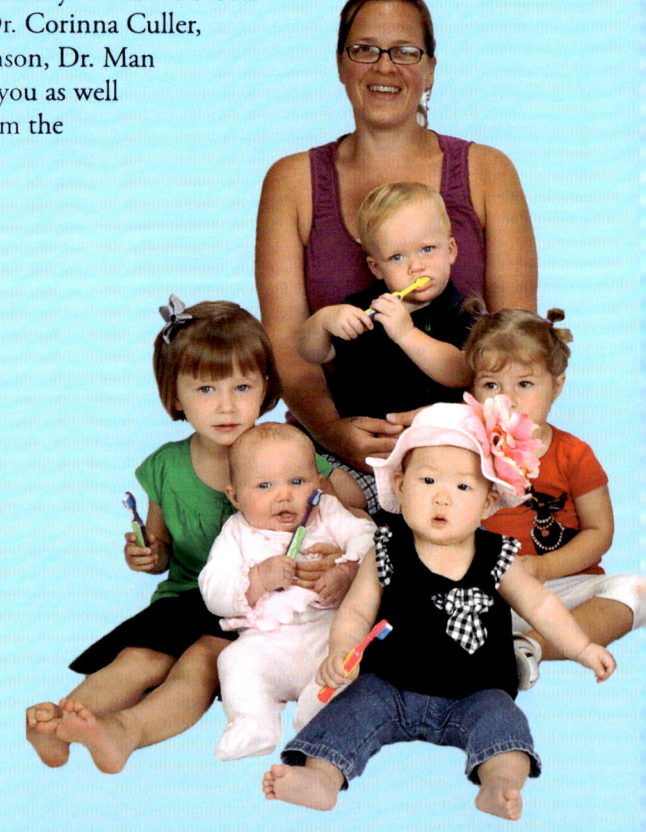

We wish to express our appreciation to Children's Dental of Waltham for allowing us to use their facility.

Our thanks to Dr. Srismitha Modem, DMD and the following families for allowing us to photograph them: the Bostroms, the Curto-Levys, the Goyals, the Rotarus, the Weis, the Wilsons, the Zeffs and the Farren-James family.

And finally, a huge thank you to Aleena (and her dad)!